I0483582

Flexibility

10 Insider Tips

Quick Ways to Become Flexible and Gain Strength

Dan C. Wilson

© 2015

© Copyright 2015 by Dan C. Wilson - All rights reserved.

This document is geared towards providing exact and reliable information in regards to the topic and issue covered. The publication is sold with the idea that the publisher is not required to render accounting, officially permitted, or otherwise, qualified services. If advice is necessary, legal or professional, a practiced individual in the profession should be ordered.

- From a Declaration of Principles which was accepted and approved equally by a Committee of the American Bar Association and a Committee of Publishers and Associations.

In no way is it legal to reproduce, duplicate, or transmit any part of this document in either electronic means or in printed format. Recording of this publication is strictly prohibited and any storage of this document is not allowed unless with written permission from the publisher. All rights reserved.

The information provided herein is stated to be truthful and consistent, in that any liability, in terms of inattention or otherwise, by any usage or abuse of any policies, processes, or directions contained within is the solitary and utter responsibility of the recipient reader. Under no circumstances will any legal responsibility or blame be held against the publisher for any reparation, damages, or monetary loss due to the information herein, either directly or indirectly.

Respective authors own all copyrights not held by the publisher.

The information herein is offered for informational purposes solely, and is universal as so. The presentation of the information is without contract or any type of guarantee assurance.

Table of Contents

Introduction

Are you struggling with getting in shape? Want to look better? Looking for ways to improve your physical results?
This book shows you how to do all three!

What you're about to discover is my unofficial guide for getting results in the gym. I'll teach you how to overcome obstacles in the gym and get you to the next level with **10 insider tips**.

Don't get lost in all the fitness books that are promising you massive muscle gains or weight loss in just a couple of days. Let's get this straight out of the way, it's **not** possible and it's also unrealistic. That being said, it can be made **easy**.

I've come across many diet plans that promise exactly the same, and to be fair it can be done. However, your body will shrimp in a very unhealthy way in a very short amount of time. Not only is this unhealthy for your body, it's also not a sticking habit that you can apply for the rest of your life, it's a *short-term solution*.

As soon as the few days or weeks are over, you will go back to your old and bad habits, and before you know it - the pounds that you've lost are already back in twice fold.

In this book we will examine common mistakes, frequently asked questions and how to approach the gym in a normal and healthy way, and more importantly how to stick with it.

My name is Dan C. Wilson and I have been involved and passionate about the sports and fitness industry for many years. Not only have I been a fitness instructor to numerous people, I have also completed many courses for being able to give you the best information and help you to overcome any health obstacle, which will sooner or later arrive in your life.

Now, why is exercising so important for us?
Surely, if your plan is to lose a certain amount of pounds then you can simply eat less and the goal will be reached... **WRONG**!

#1
Getting Back Into Shape

Not only is this a totally wrong way of thinking, it never works out the way you want it to be. Cutting down on food not only makes your body a lot weaker, it will drip your energy level below zero and you'll become an easy victim for sickness.

It's a lot easier to keep all of your current habits, and add one additional habit at a time– which is exercises. Not only will you feel weak and unhealthy when you stop eating, it will also not get you much pleasure by achieving your weight loss goal. This almost always ends up getting you frustrated and *eating more* than you did before.

I'm a big fan of doing things **slow and steady**.
As the saying goes; "*slow and steady wins the race*".

Trying to rush your achievements will only make things worse. I see it happen too often in the gym, people are trying to reach a certain amount of weight they want to lift and they end up with injuries. Next thing you know, they are not able to exercise for the next couple of weeks, they lose their habit and motivation and are never to be seen back in the gym. Instead of trying to aim for a specific goal, it is much better to track your results and simply trying to <u>improve</u> them.

Not only is this better for the long term run, you will also create a habit to keep improving yourself. People believe that going to the gym and doing the exercises is just to lose some fat and gain muscles, I totally **disagree** with that statement.

Sure, you will lose fats and gain muscles but that's usually only the first motivation for people to sign up for a subscription at the local gym. You will notice that when you are not trying to aim for a specific goal, you will start to enjoy doing exercises on a daily basis a lot more. You will see improvements, and you simply feel more energetic and healthier.

This habit will get you much further in life than gaining just a few muscles. As you keep trying to improve yourself, you will see better results in your job as well. Setting specific goals will only hold you back as they limit yourself. They don't allow you to reach the sky and beyond.

EXAMPLE

If you're a salesman in your daily life, your boss may have given you a sales target to reach at the end of the month. The next month is about to start and you have to sell 20 products during that month. You are super motivated to reach the goal as you don't want to get fired. Now, you may have had a perfect week giving you exactly the 20 sales needed for this particular month. What happens next...?

NOTHING! You have reached your goal and your boss is pleased and not asking for more, so why would you?

This is why building up a habit of trying to improve yourself is so important for you. Setting specific goals means failure. A much better approach is trying to *improve* the sales you had last month, instead of trying to reach a static 20 sales goal per month. This will not stimulate you to get better results, and you will never reach your full potential. For all we know, you may have the actual potential to reach the yearly objective within just 1 month.

I cannot stress this enough that doing exercises on a daily basis will get you much more in life than simply losing a few pounds. Cancelling the subscription as soon as you have reached your goal, just to sign up for the gym again within 6 months, and trying to reach the same goal.

By noticing improvements, and seeing what you are actually capable of without limits will give you so much more confidence. This confidence will lead you to great things in life. As you become more confident of yourself, this will reflect to everyone around you. You are less afraid to take decisions, you are not afraid to start a conversation with the girl or guy who you've been admiring for such a long time. You have the confidence to tell your boss "no".

Feeling comfortable with your body is by far the greatest feeling. When you don't feel comfortable with yourself, how can someone feel comfortable with you? We need to work on ourselves first before we can spread our confidence and happiness to others. Starting by getting into shape is **the first step** to become more self-aware, comfortable and confident about yourself.

While you continue reading this book, you will find a lot more *great tips* together with the best approaches for improvements and how to avoid common mistakes.

Let this book be a guide for you to reach the next level in your current life state. Now that you are more convinced about doing exercises and signing up for a monthly subscription at your local gym, let's move on to the next step.

#2

Thoughts on Personal Trainers

So you have finally made the decision and signed up for a subscription at the local gym. Congratulations!

Perhaps this was a long struggle for you and you haven't stopped thinking about it for the previous days, weeks or maybe even months. Feels good doesn't it?

You have achieved something which you wanted to do for such a long time. And it wasn't that hard at all. In fact, the people at the gym were more than happy to welcome you.

Being a fitness instructor in the past, I have seen so many shy and uncomfortable people come and leave. Don't ever think that the people working at the gym are just after your money. This is not a sales job, they are truly happy and willing to give you the best possible advice they can.

EXAMPLE

Have you never felt grateful, when someone asked for advice? They could have asked anyone on the world, but they decided to ask you. This probably gave you so much pleasure and surely created a smile on your face that kept you going for the rest of the day.

During my instructor career I've helped so many people. Seeing how they progress, starting to feel more comfortable, becoming happy and embracing life again is a priceless feeling. I don't have children (yet), but I can totally imagine this is what it feels like to see your child growing up and succeeding in life.

Now, as you've signed up for the subscription at your gym, you're probably wondering whether or not you should ask advice from one of the many instructors walking around.

If you're an absolute beginner then all I can say is... **YES**!
Especially, when you're totally new and unfamiliar with all the different machines. This can be very intimidating, which may result into starting to doubt your decision of signing up for the gym. <u>Don't worry about it</u>!

We've all had our first day in the gym, job, a new city, anywhere. You need to start feeling comfortable with not only the gym itself, but also the people who will be there on a daily basis. Be it the instructors or people like you, who love to work out and improve their limits.

I've seen so many great things happening in the gym that I can only tell you to *take the first step*.

If there's currently no instructor available, don't be shy to ask someone else who's working out his daily routine just like you. They are more than happy to help you out. It can happen that an instructor is currently occupied and helping somebody else, leaving you alone for a short moment. Don't be shy to start working on an exercise. People will know that you're new and unfamiliar with all the exercises, and sooner or later they will approach you to explain a few things and help you out as the instructor is occupied.

That being said, if this is the first day at the gym. Don't hesitate to ask any fitness instructor to help you out. Don't worry about being specific, it's actually much better to not have a specific goal in mind so that the instructor can give you his best advice possible.

I've had many customers come in and asking me *"what is best way to lose 10 pounds within a month?"*, because they want to be in shape when they are about to go on vacation, and will be spending a couple of days on the beach.

Asking for a very specific goal will narrow down the possibilities, and usually this leads to lower standards. I can give people various daily schedule plans to quickly lose 10 pounds. However, I really don't support approaching your goals like this. It is good to have a certain goal in mind, but <u>don't make your goal too specific</u>.

Not only does this narrow down the possibilities for the instructor, but also for *you*. Give the instructor enough space, and I can **assure** you that you will get a much better workout plan with solid advice compared to asking for a specific achievement.

Doing exercises have to become a habit that you *enjoy*, rather than seeing it as a job that you have to complete quickly and move on. That being said, as this may be your first day, don't hesitate to approach the instructor and let them know your goals.

EXAMPLE
Let's say you are a mother with 2 children, you're having a fulltime job and you would also like to spend some time with your husband and friends. You don't think you have the time to go to the gym every single day for the rest of your life. Achieving a certain goal doesn't always mean that you HAVE TO exercise on a daily basis. The instructor is aware of that, and as you explain your lifestyle and the situation that you are in, your instructor can then make a specific training plan <u>specially made for you</u>. This will *ensure* you that nothing too much is asked, and you should be able to reach your goals without seeing it as something annoying.

If you don't have a specific goal in mind, perfect!
By explaining your current situation and that you would simply like to get in shape is already *more than enough* information for an instructor to start working out something for you.

Now, for the more advanced readers out there. It's never a bad thing to ask for some advice either. Even for the more advanced athletes, who have a rough idea or maybe are even experts in their field and know what they are doing, it's *always* helpful to get insight from other people who have studied your field and most likely are advanced or experts just like you.

It doesn't have to mean that you will follow up the advice from the instructor to the letter, as you've created your own successful schedule and habits already. But for all you know, this could actually be *the little missing piece* that will set you up to the next level.

Don't struggle too long without getting results. Don't feel too arrogance to ask for advice, because you've been going to the gym for the past 5 years and you know what you're doing. Instructors will actually see this as **a great challenge**, as this doesn't happen a lot, they will be more than happy to test your abilities and give you new ideas and advice.

Whether you're an absolute beginner or more advanced, never hesitate to ask your fitness instructor to point out the right direction. Not only will this make your life much easier, you will reach your goals faster and keep improving yourself.

#3
Weekly Workout Schedule

A very common question is; *"how many times per week should I workout to notice a difference and keep improving?"*

To be fair, it depends on many factors. If your eating habits are bad, you can go to the gym all you want but *the results won't be there*. It's a good thing to look at things from a bigger overview and perspective. When you only focus on a small detail, you will lose sight of other more important factors that will improve your overall results a lot easier compared to trying to fix that one small detail.

I **always** advise creating the habit of working out at least 3 times per week.
By taking out all the other factors, I have created a small rule of thumb.

** **1-2 workout per week**: none to small improvements
** **3 workouts per week**: medium improvements
** **4-5 workouts per week**: high improvements
** **5+ workouts per week**: medium improvements

As you can see, trying to aim for 4 times per week should give you the most potential improvement possible. If you only workout once or twice per week, it has very little effect, because you don't put enough pressure and stress on your body to change.

However, do <u>not</u> mistake the more you work out, the better the results will be. Notice that when you work out more than 5 days, your results will actually *decrease*. This is because you really want to give your body enough time to rest between your workout programs. To give you an example and explain it better, let's take a look at your career.

EXAMPLE

If you keep making over hours every single day, and from time to time even work 6 or 7 days instead of 5 days, you aren't able to maintain this for a long time. Your body will start to weaken, you lose focus, you lose motivation, and at some point everything will *crash down*. You will end up with a burnout, and you are out of the routine for the next couple of weeks, or maybe months. Now, if only you had started out a bit less enthusiastic and more steady... meaning that you give a 110% for only a couple of hours every day. Chances are that you end up with **much better results** compared to the person who worked himself towards a burnout. This principle goes for everything you do in life, don't force things.

Slow and steady wins the race.

Now that you hopefully agree that you should aim for roughly 3-4 times per week, you certainly don't need to forget about all the other factors. But we will get into those at a later stage in this book.

My advice without knowing anything about your private life, including nutrition and your work schedule, would be 3 times per week. While giving you this number about how many times you should work out, it's also important to take a look at HOW you do your workout session. When I tell you that you should try and aim for going to the gym at least 3 times per week, that doesn't mean that I want you to spend 3 hours of your time every time in the gym.

It's very important to be *efficient* when you decide to spend some time in the gym. Not only will this give you the best health benefits to your body, it will also keep you motivated. Should I give you a workout schedule, which asks for 3 hours of your time every single day for the next 4 weeks then surely enough you will give up at and quit at some point.

Should I only ask for *45 minutes* of your time, chances are much higher that you are able to stick to the program. So not only is it important to consider how many times you actually go to the gym, it's also important to know how much time you are going to spend there.

In case you choose to spend 3-4 hours doing exercises in one go, then you will end up with the same situation as the burnout example on the previous page. Your body will get *the maximum and best results* when you do an <u>intense 45-60 minutes workout</u>. When you go beyond that, you will increase the chances of getting injuries and muscle soreness. Not only that, but your energy and strength level will simply decrease as well. You **cannot** keep lifting 80 pounds deadlifts for an entire hour.

If you think you simply don't have enough time to go to the gym, and that's holding you back, then now you will understand that it's very possible for every individual to start working out and getting back into shape.

I would strongly suggest to aim for at least <u>3 times per week</u>, and not spending more than **45-60 minutes** in the gym. That being said, should your lifestyle only allow 1 or 2 workout sessions per week, you should still *go for it*. Even though the results may be slightly less compared to going 3-4 times per week, there WILL be progress and improvement. Even by doing a 15 minute workout of pushups or sit-ups every day will already improve your body.

Now that you have a better understanding on how many times per week you should go to the gym, and how long you should spend your time there, let's move on and examine the other factors, such as the importance of *nutrition*.

#4
Taking Care of Nutrition

Thinking that you can get great results by going to the gym, and visit the McDonald's afterwards as a treatment for your commitment is **wrong**. Now of course I wouldn't have to tell you that and it's probably a somewhat extreme scenario, that everyone would disagree with. However, you would be surprised of how bad your current *eating habits* may actually be.

Ideally, you want food to SUPPORT you and <u>improve</u> your body, rather than the other way around and working *against* you. Knowing what you eat, and in which portions can give your results a great boost.

I have struggled with this for a fair amount of time during my life, where I was simply not seeing results even though I was spending quite some time in the gym giving a full 110%. Not noticing any improvements, regardless of how hard you work for it can be very *demotivating* and makes you question yourself.

Once I finally reached the point of becoming demotivated and slowly started to give up, I started to question myself. The last part is always a **very strong** and **important** moment in your life. I started to do more research and I started to examine my own habits. By taking a closer look to myself, I was noting everything down on paper.

Starting from the amount of sleep, what time I was waking up, how long I would wait before eating breakfast, which type of breakfast was I eating, how much time did I give my body to digest the food before going to the gym... <u>every single detail</u> of my daily life.

Now, soon enough after *weeding out* the lesser important things in my daily routine such as cleaning the dishes, I was left with my **food schedule**.

After doing thorough research and yes... even I asked for advice from various instructors, it was obvious that my way of eating was *wrong*.

However, I do want to point out that since usually it's very obvious that the things you eat is part of the issue – It's not something you actually start looking at when you decide that you want to become bigger.

Becoming bigger means simply more eating, right? No. I actually made two big mistakes and that was:

1. Eating **too much**, where most of the amount was simply stored as fat, I was also…

2. Eating the **wrong** foods. You want food to *support* your body; I was simply eating the wrong foods and the wrong amount that made me ending up working out to digest my food. It doesn't take rocket science to notice when you are doing exercises to get rid of the excessive amount of food, you won't be improving. Your body will stay in the same shape if you don't change your diet plan.

We won't be going into the very specific details, as I am actually covering a lot of nutrition facts plus a very helpful diet in one of my other books. Now, I don't want to be the self-promoting kind of person but I would highly suggest checking out the Ketogenic Diet plan.

It's not just a random diet plan that I'm asking you to check out. No, the ketogenic diet *works very well* in combination with fitness. This will keep your energy level high, and your body will use a different kind of energy source. Not only will this make you *rapidly lose weight and fat*, the recipes are very delicious at the same time!
So, if you are more interested in different kinds of diets to *support* your body, rather than working against you. I would highly suggest checking out the book below. I've left you a preview of the ketogenic diet plan at the end of this book, in case you are interested.

Ketogenic Diet: Foolproof 4 Weeks Diet Plan - Quick & Fast Ketogenic Recipes (5 BONUS Recipes)

In case you're a reader who's not interested in *losing weight*, but you actually want to <u>gain weight</u>. This book will also be very helpful for you. The recipes are natural and healthy, and where some meals are skipped – simply add a recipe to your likings.

Becoming bigger, doesn't simply mean that you should eat more and more. You don't want to get too much of fat that your body cannot process anymore. You will end up working out to just *lose* the additional fat, but as you keep adding fats – there won't be much of a progress to see.

In case you're not aware of all the different factors in fitness. I would strongly suggest to <u>just get started</u>.
I see it happening more than often that people *overthink* everything they do in life. I'm a strong believer of simply getting started, and figuring it out as I go. Trying to make everything perfect *before* you start, will not only **delay** your results, it's also a sort of **procrastination**. Embrace the fact that you will <u>never</u> be able to have the *perfect* preparation, not even after a year or two.

There will always be additional ways to improve and new things to try.

So, if you were planning to figure out a workout schedule, a food diet, different kinds of supplements, and the list goes on before you start, DON'T do it.

This will simply *delay* your improvements, and before you know it you'll end up not going anymore because it's too overwhelming.

Since you've already signed up for a monthly subscription at your local gym, **just go** and start doing some exercises. Don't think about having the right workout program, or not knowing what you are doing.

If you have asked your fitness instructor for help, then sure enough you will receive a schedule which is *specifically* designed for **your** needs. In the meantime... just explore the different machines and exercises.

Just take in mind to not overdo it. You really *don't* want to end up with an injury the day before you receive your personal training schedule.

Before you actually get started it's important to not just start right off the bat. Don't worry, I'm not suddenly saying you *shouldn't* do exercises, I'm talking about **stretching**.

#5
The Importance of Stretching

Before you get started with doing the more heavy weight lifting, or just doing cardio. It is *important* to **warm up** your body and muscles before you start. This will <u>lower</u> the chances of serious injuries. If you have already received your workout schedule from your fitness instructor, then I would simply suggest to follow what he has recommended for you. In some cases it might take a little bit longer than you were hoping for. So therefore, I feel obliged to explain you a few things about stretching and warming up your muscles. It would be a waste if you end up with a serious injury after your very first week.

It's important to be aware of the *benefits* and also the different kind of exercises you should be doing before starting your regular workout program. As with the nutrition subject, we won't be going too much in depth about all the different stretching exercise, the benefits and the things you really want to avoid.

I have covered a whole bunch about stretching techniques and dedicated a book to this subject, which I believe would be a great asset to your knowledge if you are *serious* about getting started with <u>getting in shape</u>. I've left you a preview at the end of this book together with the ketogenic diet plan, in case you are interested.

Following the book title below will redirect you to the book, which will get you started with excellent stretching exercises to avoid injuries and becoming more flexible.

<u>Stretching: Stretching Exercises for Beginners – Quick Ways to Become Flexible and Gain Strength</u>

However, more than likely your fitness instructor has not left out a good quality warm up and cooling down routine to prepare your body before starting with the more heavy lifting. So again, should your instructor already have a workout program prepared for you, then I would suggest to simply follow his instructions.

That being said, I do have to note that the Stretching book not only contains *different exercises* together with a <u>workout program</u>. On top of that you will find all the different kind of *health benefits, and things to avoid*.

Be very cautious with starting right off the bat without doing proper warming up exercises. In case you've managed to get yourself an *injury*, then read on...

#6

How to Improve when Injured

Many people are not aware of the *importance* part of stretching and preparing the muscles with a warm up. This will usually lead to muscle soreness or injuries.

EXAMPLE
You've done all the needed preparation before you start working out, you've listened closely to the advice of your instructor, and perhaps you've even read my book about *stretching* to be fully prepared. Nothing can go wrong, right? <u>Wrong</u>.

Being prepared doesn't always necessarily mean that *nothing* can go wrong anymore from this point. That being said, it doesn't even have to mean that you'll obtain an injury just by doing exercises in the gym. Perhaps you've twisted your ankle when walking down the road on your way to the supermarket to buy ingredients for one of the lovely recipes from the *ketogenic diet plan*.
Injuries can happen anywhere and at any given time. Perhaps you woke up with cramps in your leg.

Now, of course you can take measures and try to <u>minimize</u> the risks of getting an injury. Doing exercises on a regular basis will *lower the chances*, especially when doing stretches. But unfortunately they **cannot** be avoided at all times.
This isn't immediately the end of the world, should you be reading this while having an injury. Maybe you went beyond your body limits while you were doing squats, and now you can barely walk up the stairs. *Don't worry too much.*
You could've broken an arm... that doesn't right away mean that you are absolutely useless and you're out of the routine for weeks.

It's an unfortunate set back, but it shouldn't withhold you from doing exercises. Now that you are more familiar with the people working in your gym, I would first of all strongly suggest asking advice from your fitness instructor.

When we are discussing injuries, it is important to know <u>exactly</u> what we are talking about and how it happened.

How can we treat it, and speed up the process? How can you avoid getting the same injury again in the future? All this information matters when you're dealing with an injury.

Especially if you've worked yourself into an injury when doing an exercise, it is *important* to talk with your instructor about it.

Most gyms have *physical therapy* available for you, and will make you an appointment with a more experienced physiotherapist. <u>Don't worry</u> about not being able to do any exercise at all for the next few weeks.

Even though I'm not a physio expert, I've had my fair share of injuries and treatments as well. More than once it happened that I've overdone an exercise resulting into a *lower back injury*. However, as it's certainly not the most pleasurable feeling in the world, with the right amount of *determination*, you can still proceed working out and **improve** your body.

EXAMPLE

Let's assume you've broken your leg for a minute, and the next couple of weeks you *won't* be able to move your right leg.

This happened when you got into trouble while trying to impress your friends with your new Snowboard on a vacation in the snowy mountains. You struggle your way into the gym, and everybody is looking slightly confused at you as you proceed to the changing room with crutches. As it might feel a little bit strange and odd at first, are they perhaps right and it's totally *unthinkable*? **Of course not**! You can still do PLENTY of exercises. Have you not been aware of the great things like the Paralympics? People can achieve great things, even when they are MISSING body parts.

So why can't you keep doing what you are doing with an injury? Sure, I don't recommend if you are walking on crutches to start doing leg exercises. That wouldn't be a smart move for sure. However, don't see this as a setback *to train* and *improve* your biceps and triceps. You CAN train your shoulders, chest and many more parts of your body.

If you're having an injury, simply proceed by giving that particular part of your body <u>rest</u> and *focus* on other muscle parts. As I gave you an example of my silly mistakes and being able to get lower back injuries, maybe you took a guess already but it happened with deadlifts. Once I'm aware of the fact that I've worked myself into a lower back injury, I simply proceed by focusing on *different* parts of my body until the injury is <u>fully recovered</u>.

The next time you will be more cautious, but take note of the words "*the next time*". If you've gotten into an injury by doing a particular exercise, that doesn't mean you should just *skip* it the next time and trying to avoid any chance of getting the same injury again.
You should **overcome your fears**, and get on where you've had a <u>minor</u> setback.
Even though, nowadays I am *slightly* more cautious with the deadlift exercise, I am still doing it regularly on a weekly basis. And with being more cautious, I don't mean that I am lowering the weight. No! I am more cautious with my preparation, body form, and any other additional thing I can do.

As you can realize now, obtaining an injury doesn't *always* have to be a bad thing. It makes you aware of the mistakes that you made, and the next time you will do things **RIGHT**. This will <u>improve</u> your results a lot more. So learn from your mistakes, and improve them. Do NOT run away from them. Sometimes we have to learn things the hard way, but it's still a learning process where we are able to come out **stronger**.

#7
Combining Weights with Cardio

By now you've had a fair share of doing different kind of exercises, which probably have been lifting weights and doing stretches.
You don't feel very comfortable with all those massive muscled men in the weights room, and you prefer to do some cardio exercises instead.
Now I can be a twat, and tell you to stop caring about other people, but I won't.

You should do what your *heart* is telling you, and if lifting weights isn't for you, then how could you possibly stay <u>motivated</u> and keep doing the exercises on a regular basis for the next few years?

If doing cardio exercises is more appealing for you, then I'm always willing to support you. Or perhaps you are interested in *both*.

I often get the question; *"Is it possible to gain muscles AND work on your condition?"*

Yes, it's possible. But that said, you would need to try and <u>balance</u> it. You will *not* be able to create the body size of Arnold Schwarzenegger and have the speed and condition from Usain Bolt at the same time.
However, if you are interested in doing both then you can totally combine it.

In fact, there are plenty of people who are following a schedule of 2 or 3 days of weightlifting combined with 1 or 2 days of cardio exercises.
Lifting weights day after day will not improve your body on a *conditional* body a lot. And running for miles every day will not improve your *strength* in the arms a lot either. But it's *possible* to train them at the same time.

It's a common saying in the gym that you will lose your muscles when you start doing cardio. Which is **not** entirely true, it highly depends on the type of cardio that you are doing.

EXAMPLE

If you're aiming for building a muscular body, but would like to have a decent conditional level at the same time – I would *not* suggest doing high interval running. As this type of cardio is purely meant to <u>lose</u> a high amount of fats, which you don't want to lose because this will help you to GROW your muscles. Good cardio exercises while maintaining or even *improving* your muscular body are, by far on **number 1**; rowing. This cardio exercise does not only train your condition, you will also *gain* muscle improvements in your legs, as well as your arms. In case you are more of a swimming type, then this would be also a very good solution. You can even go mountain biking outside.

The trick to combine *gaining* and **improving** your muscles together with cardio exercises is to <u>not</u> go beyond your limits.

Once you start doing for example interval training, you will start burning fats, which is normally a good thing for most people BUT if you want to become **bigger**, then you definitely want to *avoid* interval sessions.

Good ways to combine strength and stamina is by doing a <u>30-45 minute</u> of *medium* cardio.

You will improve your conditional level, while at the same time you are not losing a high chunk of your fats. I won't be creating a top 10 cardio exercises for you to follow, as this highly depends on your OWN preferences.

If you're not a running type of person, then you should aim for biking or any other cardio exercise. It is <u>very</u> important to pick the exercise that *you* like doing the most.

This way you are able to keep the motivation up. If it's a pain for you every time you start your way towards the gym, then it's just a matter of time before you cancel the gym subscription.

To summarize whether you can or cannot <u>combine</u> cardio together with lifting weights; **yes, you can**. Just make sure to keep the cardio exercises on a *medium* level. If you go beyond the limits, not only will you increase the chances of injuries, your body will be very week the next day. This won't allow you to lift the heaviest weights possible.

Now, there may be some supplements that can help you...

#8

Which Supplements to Use

During my years spent in the gym, I've had a fair amount of people asking me for advice about which *supplements* they should use. There are so many out there, and they all seem to be very promising.

Let me tell you straight away, **95%** of all the supplements are not only a waste of your money, they are bad for your *health* as well.

Most supplement products are created by waste and leftover ingredients from other products, and promoted as the next best thing on the market. Bodybuilders are willing to try and consume anything when you tell them this will help to improve strength and muscles and get them to the next level.

I've never been a big fan of supplements, nor have I tried them all. And I can proudly say that my body looks perfectly, without all the unnecessary products out there. You DON'T need supplements to look strong.

However, there's **one** product that I'm a big fan of and by using this you can notice great improvements pretty much straight away, and that's creatine.

A small amount will only cost you roughly $5 or $10 and lasts for a long time (2-3 months). Not only is this *very good value* for your money, it will help you to improve your strength and muscle gain.

I've heard many stories about whey protein, and how everyone should use it.

Truth is, I have *stopped* using it a long time ago. The prices are rather high, and most people cannot even afford it. You'll be spending $50 every 2 months for a small gain, which is in discussion amongst the fitness people. Because, not only do you have to pay for the gym subscription, you want to make sure you buy the best foods out there that *support* your body, you may need to pay an extra amount of gasoline in case you have to go to the gym by car, sports outfit, shoes, and the list goes on... So why pay another hundred bucks for more supplements?

I won't go into a full depth explanation about every supplement out there, because that's not the main focus of this book, nor do I have enough experience to share my thoughts about every single supplement. There's just way too many to talk about.

If you're *new* to the gym and just started your journey of lifting weights, I recommend **not** using supplements at all. Your body doesn't need any additional help, because you first have a long way to go to even reach your *maximum* body potential. Now, when you are slightly more experienced and advanced and you feel like you hit a roadblock that prevents you from improving and lifting *heavier* amounts of weights I will recommend giving creatine a try. This product is totally natural, and will not harm your body in any way.

Now which Creatine to use?

You want to be looking for **creatine monohydrate**, this is the best form you can get and it's the most *natural* for you. I have provided a great creatine supplement below, which is also the one I'm using for years, and I'm still positive about it. I'm not receiving a single penny should you decide to buy it, so you can trust that it's totally recommended by me and I'm not asking anything in return, or simply trying to get a few extra bucks.

Optimum Nutrition Creatine Powder

If you're not familiar with creatine or supplements in general, then I would suggest buying the *lowest* amount which is 150g for only $5.03. That's only 3 cents per gram, a pretty fair deal, *right*? Plus this amount should last you at least for a **month**.

Creatine monohydrate is one of the most *well-researched* sports nutrition ingredients. It has been proven that in regular weight training, it supports muscle size, strength and power. Make sure to follow the instructions and sticking with the recommended intake per day. Suggested is 5 gram per time, mixed with water, juice or your post-workout protein shake to help you meet ambitious weight room goals.

If you decide to buy this supplement, you would still need to keep the *motivation* up. None of the supplements that you decided to buy will improve your strength with <u>doing nothing</u>. Let's take a look at ways to staying **motivated**...

#9
Staying Motivated

You've bought the needed supplements to get you to the next level, and basically got everything else needed...
You've become far more experienced and people starting to *recognize* your face in the gym. But you sense that you're losing motivation.
You've reached a certain goal, and you're not aiming for something new anymore.

We've discussed at the start of this book, that first of all that's the **wrong** approach of keeping the motivation up in the gym. However, having reached your main goal isn't the end of the world.
But what's your next goal going to be? *Exactly*, nobody knows.

Unfortunately, I don't have the Holy Grail formula for you that gives you infinite motivation. There are some methods that work for some, but are counterproductive for others and get actually more demotivated.
I've read some motivation books, and I would like to suggest taking a look at the motivation book down below. I believe it's a fair new author and he recently published a very valuable book on Amazon.
As this was for free during that time, I picked up my copy as I believe *motivation* is a strong key element in our life.
When going through this book, I found a lot of good exercises that helped me. The person seems very honest, and therefore I would *recommend* taking a look. Unfortunately, I can't provide a preview as it's not work of mine. But luckily enough, Amazon provides small previews of books before you decide to buy it.

The book will teach you ways to get fast development results and quick simple innovation techniques.

There are many *helpful* exercises which can be found in this book, that will surely keep you motivated and think about certain situations.

Another thing I would like to add from my own experience is, even though I am not very experienced with the human brain like the author Dave Chandler, what I feel what works best for me is, once I'm starting to see **progress** not only in the mirror but also on <u>paper</u>, that's what's keeping me motivated and makes me want to *push my limits*.

Now, before we move on to how to track your results and keep *pushing* yourself to reach **new** goals, let me provide you the book title for your motivation process below.

<u>Motivation: How to Get Fast Development Results, Quick Simple Innovation Techniques, Learn the Secrets of Happiness</u>

#10
How to Track Results

Once you've reached your <u>main objective</u>, it's usually hard to stay motivated as you don't have another *goal* to aim for. That's not always a bad thing.
I would strongly suggest you to keep **track** of your results, this is exactly what I am doing as well and has kept me going for years.

I get often asked *"What are good ways to track results? Could you recommend me an application for my phone?"*

I don't have advice for downloading an application for your phone, as frankly, I wouldn't even know any application at all for fitness and keeping track of it.
That being said, what I found that works best for me is by simply *noting* down everything you do in the gym.

EXAMPLE
Let's say you start your first week with a bench press of 30kg. You want to note that down. It's easy to lose track of your previous results, when you're doing a mixture of different exercises, or when you were out of the routine for a small moment. Before I started noting things down, I was pretty lost as well at some point. You <u>cannot</u> remember the weights you were using the last time, and unconsciously you are actually pushing lower weights than you did before.
You really don't want to **decrease**. I would only suggest *lowering* the weights, if you have either an <u>injury</u> or you are trying to cut in fats.

So how do I keep track of my routine? *Simple.* I've created a spreadsheet where I note down all my results of that particular workout.
If your weekly workout exists of 3 days and 5 different exercises.
<u>Write them down</u>, so that afterwards, or while you are working out your exercises you can fill in the gaps.

This makes it so much **easier** to not only keep track of your improvements, it also *stimulates* you to improve yourself every week. I've given you an example of **how I keep track** of my results on the next page, and I will explain it a bit further. Although it's quite straight forward, I usually find that simplicity works best for these kinds of things.

Week 6	
Exercise	Amount
Squats (4 sets)	27.5
Leg press (3sets)	180
Leg extensions (2 sets)	
Leg curls (3 sets)	50
Stiff leg deadlift (3 sets)	25
Standing calf raises (3 sets)	40
Seated calf raises (3 sets)	120

Quads/hamstrings

Exercise	Amount
Deadlift (3 sets)	35
Pullups (3 sets)	-
Barbell row (3 sets)	20
Dumbell row (3 sets)	20
Shrugs (3 sets)	24
Barbell Curl (3 sets)	8.25
Dumbell Incline Curl (3 sets)	14
Hammer Curl (2 sets)	16

Chest/triceps

Exercise	Amount
Bench Press (3 sets)	27.5
Incline dumbell press (3 sets)	18
Dips (2 sets)	0
Military press (3 sets)	8.25
Side laterals (2 sets)	14
Rear laterals (2 sets)	14
Skullcrushers (3 sets)	16
Nieuwe triceps (3 sets)	12

Chest/Shoulder/Tricep

This was a couple of years ago, when I just started again. As you can see, this was the 6th week after being out of routine for quite some time.
Now what can we see here? My week existed out of 3 *different* workouts.

** On the first day of the week, I was aiming for **improving** my legs.
** The 2nd day was focused on my chest and triceps.
** The 3rd day was working out on my chest, shoulders and triceps.
Do note that these workouts wouldn't last more than 45 minutes per day.

Now in the middle, I have listed down every single exercise I was doing at that particular time during the 6th week. I even included *how many* sets I was doing, this was based on repetitions of 10.
Lastly, in the "amount" column, I took the weight in kilograms.

Note that my way of calculating is taking 1 side of the bar and *only* counting the weights of that one side. Some people might calculate 25kg on 1 side of the bar, and then multiply it by 2, plus adding the 20kg bar on top to make the number look bigger.
I try to keep things **simple**, as I don't want to end up doing maths in the gym.

Week 8	
Exercise	Amount
Quads/hamstrings	
Squats (4 sets)	
Leg press (3sets)	200
Leg extensions (2 sets)	75
Leg curls (3 sets)	55
Stiff leg deadlift (3 sets)	
Standing calf raises (3 sets)	45
Seated calf raises (3 sets)	130
Chest/triceps	
Deadlift (3 sets)	
Pullups (3 sets)	
Barbell row (3 sets)	22.5
Dumbell row (3 sets)	
Shrugs (3 sets)	26
Barbell Curl (3 sets)	11.25
Dumbell Incline Curl (3 sets)	
Hammer Curl (2 sets)	
Chest/Shoulder/Tricep	
Bench Press (3 sets)	30
Incline dumbell press (3 sets)	20
Dips (2 sets)	
Military press (3 sets)	
Side laterals (2 sets)	
Rear laterals (2 sets)	
Skullcrushers (3 sets)	18
Nieuwe triceps (3 sets)	

What do the colors exactly mean?
When you compare this picture of my 8th week with the previous 6th week, you'll notice that everything except the amount was the same.

Even though most numbers are colored in red, some numbers have actually been improved compared to 2 weeks ago.
Let me explain the colors. When you start noting things down during your first week, every cell is **blank**.
As you go on and fill out the numbers, you will arrive in your 2nd week. This is where you grab the paint bucket. I'm ALWAYS trying to improve results from the previous week. When I succeed to do this, I color it in **green** – this way I can see there was improvement.
In case I haven't improved the amount in the following up week, I leave it **blank**. However, when I fail to increase it in the 3rd week, I'm going to paint it **red**.

So after a couple of weeks, you will see blank, green and red cells.
Once they become red on my screen, I am going to **force** myself to paint them green the next time. So far, this strategy has worked out wonders for me and allows me to push towards my limits.

Should you have different methods, please share them, by leaving behind a review! I'm always willing to try out new things.

Summarize

There you go! These are my **10 insider tips** for getting back into shape and staying there. Just follow this plan and I can <u>assure</u> you that you'll see improvements faster than you thought.

So now it's time for you to head out to the gym...

#1 - Getting Back Into Shape

Start out slow and steady. Remember that slow and steady wins the race. Don't try to rush your journey into getting back into shape. This will only lead to disappointment and delays your progress.

#2 - Thoughts on Personal Trainers

Never think that instructors have nothing to offer to you. Whether you're a beginner or advanced, don't hesitate asking for advice when you're struggling.

#3 - Weekly Workout Schedule

Remember the rule of thumb. Try to aim for working out at least 3-4 times per week to get the best possible results. Working out more will be counterproductive.

#4 - Taking Care of Nutrition

The importance of nutrition is tremendous. Make sure that the foods you consume are *supporting* you. You don't want your nutrition working <u>against</u> you. Please check out the **Ketogenic Diet** at the end of this book.

#5 - The Importance of Stretching

Doing proper stretches before and after your workout will decrease your chances of getting *injuries*. Don't skip stretching to save time. You will pay for it in the end. You'll find a preview of the **Stretching Exercises** in the end of the book.

#6 - How to Improve Being Injured

Being injured doesn't mean that you can't improve your body. Focus on different parts of your body, and make sure that you give your injury enough rest for full recovery.

#7 - Combining Weights with Cardio

It's a common question, and yes, you CAN combine it. Try to find the right balance to work on your muscles and conditioning. Don't overdo either of them.

#8 - Which Supplements to Use

Beginner's shouldn't think about supplements at all. Once you feel like you've hit a roadblock, please refer to the creatine supplement I've provided you.

#9 - Staying Motivated

Staying motivated plays a big role in getting results. Make sure to check out the book I've provided you, it has lots of great tips. Not only to stay motivated in the gym, but everything else you do in life!

#10 - How to Track Results

Find something that works for you. If you're new, I recommend using the spreadsheet example that I'm still using today. *Simplicity* is usually best.

This checklist is broken down into an easy-to-manage process. Take it one step at a time and it won't be long until you're back into shape again.

All you have to do is take _action_.

You'll still need to work for it, but you can make it easier for yourself. Getting back into shape doesn't always have to be a real struggle and painful. Following my 10 insider tips, should get you way ahead of the rest.

I hope you have found some of the answers you were looking for, and you're absolutely read getting to the next level. All the information I have provided in the **10 insider tips** are through own experience. You now have my best recommendations and advice, that should get you to where I am today.

Finally, if you enjoyed reading this book or have any feedback suggestions, then I would kindly ask you to leave a _review_ behind on **Amazon**. Should you have suggestions for a subject in the future which you want to explore further, please let me know through the review button as well. It would be greatly appreciated by the community!

Thank you very much and I wish you all the luck towards your next goal.

Dan C. Wilson

About the author

It has been my passion and hobby to increase vitality and how to become the strongest and best version of yourself since 2009. The goals of my books are simple, it is to share powerful ideas that help us all to become stronger, healthier, more flexible in every way possible. Building strength and becoming the strongest version of yourself goes far beyond lifting heavy weights and growing muscle.

My books are all about having more vitality, flexibility, health, building better relationships, creating an attractive body, nutrition and abundance. In case you want to reach your full human potential on both mentally and physically aspect and become a strong and healthy looking person, who feels amazing every day and is respected and admired by friends, family and strangers, then you are definitely in the right place here.

It is my goal to help as many people as possible. That having said, in case I can change the life of one person and make that one person feel better and more successful in life, I have reached my goal. We are all in this together! You, me and everyone else in our community. Together we will work hard and spread the message of changing lives and make our surroundings stronger and healthier. We will create a healthier and stronger world!

Dan C. Wilson

Other books by Dan C. Wilson

Stretching: Stretching Exercises for Beginners – Quick Ways to Become Flexible and Gain Strength
By Dan C. Wilson (Author)

Free Bonus Book Included !

Find the benefits of stretching here! Proven programs and exercises to improve muscle flexibility and to avoid or recover injuries

You feel there is more to achieve with your body, but you don't know where to start. Everybody around you in the gym is making steps forward, except you. Every day when you look in the mirror you cannot see any results. How come no matter how hard you try, there is no progress at all?

This book will give you all the information you need to accomplish the maximum flexibility permitted by your body. You will learn the importance of understanding the benefits of stretching and why we should use them more often in our daily life.

All the information provided to you in this book are through own experience as well as a high amount of research on the stretching topic to being able to only give you the best recommendations and suggestions out there. With the information of this book, you should be able to accomplish your maximum flexibility and strength permitted by your body structure.

Take action today and make the first step towards your success by downloading this book "Stretching Exercises for Beginners – Quick Ways to Become Flexible and Gain Strength".

Preview of "Stretching: Stretching Exercises for Beginners – Quick Ways to Become Flexible and Gain Strength".

Chapter 1:
Benefits of Stretching

As with every subject that you are new to, it's always recommendable to understand the benefits and get yourself a bit more familiar about the subject. Don't worry, we'll get to the exercises when we've examined the importance of stretching. It's something we often neglect during our daily busy life, and therefore I'd like to create more awareness of this subject by handing out this book to the world. Basically, every single movement that you make, whether it's a significant movement or a tiny one will require moving a part of your body towards a point where your joint has to be slightly increased will be called a stretching exercise.

I have listed down below some of the benefits of stretching for you.

- ✓ Great muscular flexibility.
- ✓ Reduced injuries and pains – Use light stretches if the pain prevails.
- ✓ Improved muscular strength, flexibility and stamina – The benefit depends on the degree of how much stress you put on your muscle. For gaining more strength, medium or heavy stretches are recommended.
- ✓ Improved body posture and self image.
- ✓ Prevention of back problems.

Having an improved flexibility will bring great benefits, as you've noticed in the list above. It's a very common practice, especially in the Mediterranean region and parts of Asia. By practicing various stretching exercises on a regular basis, you will help to reduce the risk of getting injuries and muscle pains. As you become more experienced and your body has become familiar with the exercises, you'll start to become a lot more efficient when performing physical activities. Should I had to explain all the great benefits and positive reactions to your body in just 4 words, I'd describe it as "improve quality of life". Ease in body movements will be provided for your everyday activities. Even the simplest tasks such as bending over to pick up something off the floor, will be accomplished far easier, faster, better and healthier when you're body has an improved flexibility..

I'd recommend for any person out there, whether you're an athlete or a beginner, to follow a stretching program. The great benefits that you'll gain from it are worth the slight effort and time that you've put into it. Recent research studies on various injuries have shown that people with low flexibility have a highly increased chance of muscle injuries. However, don't confuse this with performing stretching exercises <u>before</u> your physical activity. The flexibility required for a lower chance of getting injuries came from following a stretch training for a certain amount of weeks. By following a stretch training you will not only increase your body endurance and strength, but moreover has been reported that you'll increase your flexibility.

Before we're getting started I'd like to hand out a couple of tips to you. The most important one is by far including the major muscle groups into your workout schedule. Personally, I've created a rule of thumb to perform at least two exercises per every muscle group. It's always recommendable to start off light as part of your warm-up and slowly progress towards more heavier exercises to avoid injuries.

After you've finished your workout routine, don't run towards the showers just yet. It is suggested to do a proper warm-up but also a cool-down once you've finished your routine. This can be done the same way as the warm-up. Should your muscles be sore after your exercises, try to use only light stretches ranging from two to three times. Should your muscle soreness or injury persist for several days, then I recommend to continue using light stretches only. It is very important to give your muscles enough rest to recover, instead of forcing it.

1.1
Know your Limits

Now that we know the many great benefits that stretching has to offer, it is also important to know your limits and what to avoid. We'll start focusing on the primary part of any workout program, knowing your limits. Working out has to be something that you should enjoy and look forward to. If you don't find any pleasure in implementing it into your daily life, then how are you supposed to stick to a habit that you dislike?

It can be the first thing you do in the morning when you wake up, or in the evening when you finished your working shift. Times may come where you'll be experiencing slight muscle soreness while you're performing an exercise or the next day. This is all fine, but keep in mind that the pain shouldn't be a type of pain that prevents you from doing your normal physical activities.

The same theory goes for stretching. Stretching properly before, during and after a workout session, you will definitely decrease the chances of obtaining some serious injuries and you will avoid muscle soreness and pains.

It is therefore extremely important to know your body limits. Stretching is an activity that should improve your body stamina, rather than causing you pain. Stretching was invented to avoid pain and become more flexible. It might happen that you feel a small mild tension when you stretch, do not worry as this is just a temporary feeling from your body stiffness. Should it happen that you feel pain beyond this, then you've overdone it and it's necessary to lower down the tense level of your exercises.

Should you feel pain during stretching, this means that your body has employed its defense mechanism – the stretch reflex. How exactly do you trigger your defense mechanism? When you're performing stretching exercises and you stretch your muscles towards the level where you start feeling "pain". Our bodies have been evolved over the years and created safety measures to reduce the risk of harming your muscles and tendons with possible damage. The defense mechanism, that we call the stretch reflex, is a protection of your muscles. There may come times where you are too excited to stretch your muscles and tendons beyond their limits. Luckily, our stretch reflex will try and prevent this from happening. Although we have a great mechanism, you should never try and force your body beyond the limits. You will risk causing serious damage to your muscle tissues, tendons and ligaments.

Calisthenics: Female Body Workouts - Bodyweight Training and Movements
by Dan C. Wilson (Author)

Free Bonus Book Included !

Shape Your Female Body Without Weights and Dieting In Only a Few Days
You know you need to take action and start working on your female shape, but you don't really know where or how to start. Most information is too advanced, takes too much time, seem too extreme, or they just throw you in the middle of a gym where you don't even want to be. There has to be an easier way.

Discover and experience how EASY it is to build a perfect female body shape, without paying for any gym subscription or machines! All you need to do is follow the exercises and workouts that I'm handing out to you in this book. Getting a great female shape is slightly more complex than simply saying "exercise every day". And you know this as well.

The Real Struggle is Not Having the Knowledge and Experience

Most people have the desire and capacity to exercise, but something always prevents them from starting. Don't bother trying to find a partner for the gym, don't even bother paying for the gym! Sooner or later your partner will drop out, and you're left on your own...

Without the right knowledge, you won't see a lot of progress. This can be very demotivating. I've been a former Gym Instructor, and I know the daily struggle people go through when trying to progress, whether it's beginners or more advanced people. I've seen it all.

My new book Calisthenics for Women will help you to identify the best weight-free and costless exercises that will continually shape your female body. The exercises and workouts are through experience as well as thorough research and advice from other experts. Stop what you are doing, and gain knowledge that most people don't have. This book will help you experience a personal breakthrough.

Introducing: Calisthenics for Women: Female Body Workouts - Bodyweight Training and Movements - Proven Butt Workout

This book includes sections on:
- How to determine what workout routine works for women
- Getting you Started
- Beginner and Intermediate Workouts
- The BEST Calisthenics Exercises
- Proven Female Butt Workout
- Diets and Stretching Exercises
- And much, much more!

It's time to stop worrying about all the small details that has to be done before you get started. You can improve your health and build your perfect female shape as you go. This book will guide you through every exercise and workout routine to get you the best results and making you achieve your goals and dreams.

Chapter 1:
Getting Started

This book is not about the concept and definition of calisthenics, so let's get started. But wait... **How** do we get started? Don't worry! The beauty of calisthenics is that you have absolute <u>freedom</u>. You don't need to buy fancy workout equipment or getting a gym subscription to get you started. Calisthenics is for **everyone, anywhere and anytime**.

That being said, absolute freedom doesn't always work out great for everyone. Especially if you're a beginner and you have no idea where to start or how to do things the **right** way. In general too much of anything is usually a bad thing, that can be the same with calisthenics. Too much freedom will result into confusion as there's no strict playground or time schedule. Especially if you're new to something, it's good to have a <u>guideline</u> that you can follow. In this book I'll hand you these guidelines so that you can get started and make adjustments as you become more experienced. Let this book be my unofficial guide for women to build strength and gain knowledge.

Let's not get too excited and overload our bodies with too many different exercises. We will start with the basics and slowly add more. If you've been neglecting sports for quite a while, don't fool yourself that you'll be able to start doing muscle-ups right off the bat after a year or two without any exercises.

First of all you need to make your body stronger by starting with the basic exercises. Getting familiar and stronger with the basic exercises such as push-ups, dips, pull-ups and squats is the most **important** part. All the more advanced exercises are a variation or combination of the basic exercises.

So getting the basics right will get you a long way.

In the 21st century, nowadays everybody is looking for shortcuts, secrets or magic supplements for reaching the goal faster and easier. Basically, we all like to do less and achieve **more**. The truth is, there are no healthy and natural shortcuts for your body. Although, I will share <u>FOUR</u> secrets with you about calisthenics, to build strength and keeping the right **female** shapes.

** **1.** Be <u>patient</u>. Building your body into a better shape and gaining more power and strength takes time. Don't expect to turn into a superwoman overnight. Set **short term** and **small goals** to keep the motivation up, setting goals such as losing 30 kilogram is too significant and will be too far away. Cut your goals into smaller pieces, it shouldn't be a short term commitment but a <u>lifestyle</u>!

** **2**. Full body range motion. Doing things the incorrect way won't get you great results. I can't stress enough how **important** it is to perform the exercises the right way. Always be aware of your body form and making the full range of motion. While performing your repetitions try to control your body throughout the whole exercise. It will make a HUGE difference in noticing results and success or simply wasting your time. Being able to perform 5 full motion range of push-ups is way better for your body to adapt in the **right** shape instead of doing 10 sloppy repetitions, just for the sake of the number. Become committed to a <u>clean form</u> and your body will shape and adapt itself to something **beautiful**.

** 3. Female body shape. Don't add too **many** weight or extra repetitions. If you want your body to stay in shape, don't overdo your workout program. You want to make sure that you're keeping the intensity <u>high</u> so that your body will burn fats, but try avoiding adding too much weight on top of your own bodyweight. More repetitions, more sets and more weight will grow your body stronger faster but also bigger.

** 4. Nutrition. Bodybuilders love consuming food. Consuming excessive food will make your body grow. Stick to a **diet** that's working for you and avoid making your gut microbes working against you. For a good calisthenics diet that supports your body, please refer to my <u>Microbiome diet plan</u>.

<u>Microbiome Diet: 75 Best Selected Recipes to Improve your Gut Microbes and Boost Your Metabolism for Permanent Weight Loss</u>

Keep those 4 secrets in mind and I can <u>assure</u> you that you will see great **results** without becoming too big and muscled!

www.ingramcontent.com/pod-product-compliance
Lightning Source LLC
Chambersburg PA
CBHW021444170526
45164CB00001B/387